LOSING WEIGHT THROUGH SELF-HYPNOSIS

HARNESSING THE POWER OF SELF-HYPNOSIS FOR EFFECTIVE WEIGHT LOSS

Dianne Lewis

only. All effort has been executed to present accurate, up to date, reliable, complete information. No warranties of any kind are declared or implied. Readers acknowledge that the author is not engaged in the rendering of legal, financial, medical or professional advice. The content within this book has been derived from various sources. Please consult a licensed professional before attempting any techniques outlined in this book.

By reading this document, the reader agrees that under no circumstances is the author responsible for any losses, direct or indirect, that are incurred as a result of the use of the information contained within this document, including, but not limited to, errors, omissions, or inaccuracies.

INTRODUCTION TO SELF-HYPNOSIS FOR WEIGHT LOSS

Many people struggle to lose weight despite the overwhelming amount of products on the market. There are numerous quick fixes and solutions that are often ineffective. Diet plans, workout routines, weight-loss supplements, and other products are available everywhere. Each product claims that it can help you achieve an improved physique. But what would you say if we told you that the answer to weight loss was right in front of your eyes? There is an unutilized but highly effective tool that can completely change the way of losing those stubborn kilos. It's called self-hypnosis.

DEFINITION AND EXPLANATION OF SELF-HYPNOSIS

Self-hypnosis involves creating an altered state of consciousness within yourself, where you detach from your immediate surroundings, centering your attention on inner experiences like emotions, thoughts, or mental imagery.

In this process, you guide your mind into a highly focused and suggestible state, allowing you to make imagined scenarios feel exceptionally real.

Think of self-hypnosis as a form of meditation that you can intentionally access, making it a powerful tool for personal growth and therapeutic purposes. During self-hypnosis, you can provide suggestions to your own subconscious mind, both verbally and through mental imagery, to work toward specific goals. The soothing nature of self-hypnosis makes it a valuable self-help technique.

It's important to understand that self-hypnosis won't perform miracles or turn the impossible into reality, but it can help you gain insight into what's realistically achievable for you.

BENEFITS OF USING SELF-HYPNOSIS FOR WEIGHT LOSS

Self-hypnosis has quickly become an invaluable asset when it comes to weight loss. The combination of diet and exercise regimens with self-hypnosis offers numerous advantages beyond what has traditionally been available before. These pages explore the transformative potential of self-hypnosis, providing you with a key to unlocking lasting success on your journey toward healthier living. Once you begin practicing self-hypnosis, you'll realize its profound influence over your motivation, giving you the strength and drive needed to reach your weight-loss goals. Self-hypnosis also gives you increased self-control that enables you to resist temptations more easily while making healthier decisions without effort. By harnessing the power of suggestion and tapping into the latent potential of your subconscious mind, you'll find yourself not only losing weight but also freeing yourself of limiting beliefs that have held you back. Take this journey and experience extraordinary transformation through self-hypnosis for sustainable, lifelong weight-loss success.

CHAPTER 1: UNDERSTANDING THE SUBCONSCIOUS MIND AND WEIGHT

The Role of Subconscious Beliefs and Programming

Your belief systems function like subconscious programs, silently shaping your thoughts and actions. Understanding belief systems is vital for unraveling the inner workings of your mind.

These belief systems reside in your subconscious mind, acting as the driving force behind your behaviors. Picture your subconscious as a garden, and these beliefs as the plants that thrive there. Beliefs take root when a new idea embeds itself in the fertile soil of your subconscious. Your conscious mind serves as the gatekeeper, filtering ideas from trusted sources and through repetition. Beliefs germinate when these concepts infiltrate your subconscious, eventually forming a self-reinforcing cycle.

The ease of belief transformation depends on their tenure in your subconscious. Childhood beliefs are more resistant to change than those formed later in life. Reflect upon the beliefs in your mental garden, identify their sources, and consider if they align with your aspirations. If not, it's time to cultivate the beliefs you desire.

In parallel, your subconscious mind exerts profound influence over your life, governing your choices, lifestyle, and reactions to stress. Operating beneath your conscious awareness, it soaks in information, forming early, unchallenged beliefs that can hinder you as an adult. Reprogramming your subconscious mind is the key to overcoming these obstacles.

Although the transformation takes time, it manifests as increased confidence, a willingness to take risks, inner peace, and exciting goals. Consistency and persistence in reprogramming your subconscious mind are essential, as these changes hold lifelong and powerful impacts.

SCIENTIFIC RESEARCH ON THE SUBCONSCIOUS MIND AND WEIGHT

Science has shown that weight loss can be intimately connected with our subconscious mind. According to studies, hypnotherapy was found effective at helping individuals lose weight through subliminal messages that influence eating behavior in favor of healthier habits. Mindfulness techniques as well as subconscious reprogramming techniques like affirmations or visualization have proven effective in weight-loss interventions; individuals may respond differently, but all studies indicate the relevance of the subconscious in weight-loss interventions.

CHAPTER 2: SCIENCE OF SELF-HYPNOSIS

Psychological Principles Behind Self-Hypnosis

Self-hypnosis is an effective weight-loss technique that applies psychological principles such as suggestion, focused attention, and subconscious mind power to reframe people's views about food and exercise in favor of healthier alternatives. By making suggestions to the body through self-hypnosis, people can alter their beliefs about both eating and physical exercise to create healthier lifestyle choices and attitudes toward both. Self-hypnosis uses focused attention to quiet the conscious mind and gain access to the subconscious, where habits reside, to alter behavior through visualization and relaxation techniques. Visualization creates mental images of success in weight-loss goals, while relaxation aids stress reduction and promotes emotional coping mechanisms. Self-hypnosis can be an excellent complement to leading a healthier lifestyle.

NEUROSCIENCE AND BRAINWAVE PATTERNS DURING SELF-HYPNOSIS

Self-hypnosis involves shifting brainwaves away from beta waves toward alpha and theta patterns, inducing relaxation and increasing suggestibility. Beta waves indicate alertness, while alpha waves signal calmness. Self-hypnosis techniques like deep breathing or visualization can help transition you from beta waves to alpha and theta waves, providing greater receptivity for positive suggestions or therapeutic interventions as well as relaxation and stress reduction. Focus shifting promotes relaxation while tension diminishes, creating an atmosphere of tranquility. Self-hypnosis can use altered brainwaves for personal growth while decreasing stress.

STUDIES AND EVIDENCE SUPPORTING THE EFFECTIVENESS OF SELF-HYPNOSIS

Hypnosis, an ancient mind-body treatment method, has experienced a recent revival and has shown promise in treating various physiological and psychological problems such as stress, pain, and psychosomatic disorders.

A recent survey conducted by the Neurogastroenterology Unit at Wythenshawe Hospital in Manchester, UK across 31 countries sheds light on how clinical hypnosis is practiced today. Stress reduction, self-esteem enhancement, surgery preparation, anxiety intervention, mindfulness facilitation, labor, and childbirth were found to be highly successful applications, with over 70% of respondents approving of them (Palsson et al., 2023).

CHAPTER 3: TECHNIQUES AND APPROACHES TO SELF-HYPNOSIS

Visualization and Imagery Techniques

Visualization can be an extremely effective method for programming the subconscious mind. By visualizing vivid mental images of what you desire as your goal outcome, visualization allows access to this part of the mind where habits and beliefs reside. Visualization's emotional effect makes it particularly potent; engaging feelings, reinforcing positive beliefs, and increasing self-confidence all at the same time are powerful drivers for change. Relaxation techniques such as sensory engagement or repetition may assist vivid imagery. Use a positive script written in the present tense and create an atmosphere of relaxation when engaging in visualization with self-hypnosis. Visualization should engage both physical and emotional responses for lasting change; consistent practice of this method will lead to positive shifts in thoughts, behaviors, and life outcomes

DIANNE LEWIS

over time.

SUGGESTION AND AFFIRMATION METHODS

Positive affirmations are an effective tool to combat harmful beliefs and thought patterns, especially for shifting them toward desired results. For optimal effectiveness, successful affirmation practices use specific, positive language that empowers you and helps direct the mind in the desired path. To maximize affirmation practices and ensure their success, your goals should be clearly laid out, using present tense with personal pronouns when possible and visualizing images during self-hypnosis sessions, as this will engage your subconscious, allowing positive thought patterns to take root and create lasting changes within you. Patience, consistency, and repetition are keys to successfully programming your subconscious with affirmations and self-hypnosis techniques combined.

SELF-HYPNOSIS SCRIPTS AND RECORDINGS

Self-hypnosis is a potent tool for self-enhancement and personal metamorphosis, consisting of four fundamental components: induction, deepening, subject, and awakening.

- The induction establishes the framework for relaxation and centers your attention. It should involve techniques that soothe the body and mind, often encompassing profound respiration, visualization, or progressive muscle relaxation. The objective is to shift your awareness from the external world to your inner thoughts and experiences.

- Deepening procedures are employed to further relax and prime your consciousness for the hypnotic state. Deepening scripts can incorporate suggestions for descending a staircase, entering a tranquil garden, or riding an elevator. These allegorical elements deepen your trance-like condition, making you more amenable to the forthcoming suggestions.

- The core of self-hypnosis, the subject segment, is where you tackle the specific issue or goal you desire to work on. Whether it involves boosting self-assurance, conquering a phobia, or refining your sleep, the subject script should offer constructive and empowering suggestions that align with your aims. This represents the essence of the self-hypnosis session, and it is imperative to thoughtfully craft the language and imagery for optimum effectiveness.

- An awakening script is indispensable to gently guide you back to full alertness. It might encompass a countdown from 10 to 1 or a simple directive to open your eyes. This section ensures your transition from the hypnotic state and reverts to your customary state of consciousness, leaving you feeling revitalized and reinvigorated.

When constructing or choosing self-hypnosis scripts and recordings, it's essential to individualize each component according to your distinctive objectives and inclinations.

CHAPTER 4: PREPARING FOR SELF-HYPNOSIS

Creating a Calm and Conducive Environment

Creating an ideal environment for self-hypnosis is crucial to its success. A relaxing setting will reduce distractions and facilitate deep relaxation while setting clear goals and intentions will give direction to the subconscious mind, increase motivation, and allow tracking progress. To master self-hypnosis successfully, regular practice should help promote relaxation, reinforce desired change, and adapt to goals that develop over time. When combined, these three components allow individuals to access their subconscious minds for personal development and behavior change.

SETTING GOALS AND INTENTIONS FOR SELF-HYPNOSIS

Setting goals is pivotal to self-hypnosis and weight loss. They provide guidance and motivation, and having specific time-bound targets, such as losing 20 pounds in six months, provides clarity and motivation. By setting smaller milestones and measuring metrics such as weight or energy level, it is easier to monitor your progress. Positive affirmations are also key; to maximize their effects, they are best used in the present, visualizing success while remaining optimistic. Self-hypnosis relies heavily on positive affirmations to reinforce your belief in reaching your goals and improving health. Affirmations can serve as the cornerstone of self-hypnosis, giving it strength and credibility as a method for weight loss and transformation by aligning positive intention with goal setting.

DEVELOPING A SELF-HYPNOSIS ROUTINE

In addition to goals, adhering to a schedule can play a major role in creating an effective self-hypnosis program. Begin with 15-to-30-minute sessions lasting three or four times weekly and gradually build them up over time. Start with deep breathing exercises and progressive muscle relaxation to promote unwinding, use positive affirmations or guided recordings/apps when appropriate for visualizing what your desired result would look like, keep a progress journal, adjust techniques when necessary, and keep track of changes over time. Seek professional advice for complex matters that require assistance. Eventually, your self-hypnosis skills will transform over time so do be persistent, patiently working toward more complex, deeply rooted issues.

CHAPTER 5: IMPLEMENTING SELF-HYPNOSIS FOR WEIGHT LOSS

Identifying Specific Weight-Loss Goals

Specific weight-loss goals are fundamental to reaching success in the weight-loss journey. They provide clarity, motivation, and measurability—three essential ingredients of progress. Using specific goals such as "I want to lose 20 pounds in six months" sharpens focus and creates accountability on your journey forward. Convert a grand goal into manageable milestones while taking into account your lifestyle. Self-hypnosis provides additional motivation by aiding the visualization of success. Envision yourself reaching your target weight through self-hypnosis sessions by altering your subconscious mind and remaining flexible along the way. Patience and kindness toward yourself will be essential on this gradual weight-loss journey. Remember it takes time, but with clear goals and consistency, you are bound to succeed. Self-compassion should help increase your chances of success while you treat yourself gently along the way!

24

CREATING PERSONALIZED SELF-HYPNOSIS SCRIPTS

Remember that self-hypnosis is a highly individualized practice, and the more your scripts align with your personal preferences, the more effective and transformative your self-hypnosis experience will be. By personalizing each step while adhering to the core principles, you can harness the full potential of self-hypnosis for your personal growth and empowerment.

- Begin by selecting an **induction** method that speaks to you. Whether it's focusing on deep breaths, imagining a serene place, or any other relaxation technique, choose what resonates with you. This initial step should feel calming and soothing to your individual preferences.

- Customize your **deepening** segment to match your personal inclinations for relaxation. If a forest scene or an ocean setting resonates with you more than a staircase descent, incorporate these visuals. The aim is to deepen your hypnotic state using metaphors that personally resonate.

- Tailor the **subject** portion to your specific objectives. Use language that speaks directly to your goals, desires, and challenges. Whether it's boosting self-esteem, overcoming a specific fear, or enhancing your well-being, the suggestions in this segment should be deeply personal.

- As you conclude your self-hypnosis session, the **awakening** script should guide you back to full alertness in a way that feels right to you. Whether it's counting down from a number that holds personal significance or using words that resonate with your sense of renewal, this phase should be uniquely yours.

INTEGRATING SELF-HYPNOSIS WITH OTHER WEIGHT-LOSS STRATEGIES

Psychological factors, including mood disorders and stress, have a substantial influence on eating behaviors and weight gain. Addressing these aspects along with other weight-loss strategies is a must to combat obesity; cognitive-behavioral therapy (CBT) plays a big part in this regard, specifically in changing thought patterns and behaviors related to food intake.

Complementary approaches like self-hypnosis and mindfulness can supplement weight-loss programs by targeting dysfunctional eating behaviors, increasing self-motivation, and controlling stimuli more effectively. Pairing these techniques with traditional weight-loss approaches may lead to more comprehensive and sustainable results:

- Self-hypnosis can reinforce positive beliefs about healthy eating habits, making it easier to keep a balanced diet. Meanwhile, mindfulness helps develop awareness of hunger and fullness cues as part of portion control strategies.

- Self-hypnosis can boost motivation for exercise, creating a positive attitude toward physical activity. Incorporating mindfulness techniques during workouts deepens the mind-body connection for an enhanced experience during fitness regimes.

- Hypnosis can enhance nutritional education by reinforcing the importance of fueling our bodies with nutritious foods.

- Integrating self-hypnosis with support groups or cognitive behavioral therapy sessions provides a sense of community while providing extra tools for controlling emotional eating and stress management.

- Mindfulness practices work beautifully alongside self-monitoring routines to promote conscious food choices and increase longevity.

- Mindful meditation combined with self-hypnosis to reduce stress-related eating can provide a holistic approach to lifestyle modifications.

CHAPTER 6: OVERCOMING EMOTIONAL EATING AND CRAVINGS

Understanding the Emotional Triggers of Overeating

Emotional eating, an increasingly prevalent behavior, stems from an association between emotions and food consumption. Stressful situations tend to induce overeating due to cortisol-increasing appetite; comfort foods provide temporary solace during times of tension, while mindless snacking brings relief and stimulation through food consumption. Boredom leads many people down this path of emotional eating as an escape mechanism—something most don't realize they do until later! Negative emotions such as sadness or frustration may trigger cravings for comfort foods, while social settings or celebrations often compel individuals to indulge in excess eating in an attempt to fit in or bond through food. Childhood associations of sweet treats as rewards often remain with adults into adulthood. Psychological factors associated with emotional eating include being unaware, using food as a coping mechanism, and repeating patterns of eating. Solutions include journaling, mindfulness meditation, and emotional regulation programs as well as professional support that provides tools to manage emotional eating.

USING SELF-HYPNOSIS TO CHANGE EMOTIONAL RESPONSES TO FOOD

Self-hypnosis can help change emotional reactions to food and lead to healthier eating habits by tapping into the subconscious mind's suggestibility during relaxation. At first, one needs to identify emotional triggers like stress or boredom that lead them toward overeating; self-hypnosis provides solutions for changing emotional triggers that cause overeating and overindulgence. Self-hypnosis employing positive affirmations and visualization is used to reprogram one's subconscious and influence behavior changes in relation to food choices, portion control, and emotional triggers without resorting to food as a solution. Individuals visualize making healthier food selections while experiencing full satisfaction from smaller portions and managing emotional triggers without resorting to food as a solution. Techniques for relieving and managing negative emotions are also included, with consistent practice being essential to creating lasting change and professional assistance helping ensure maximum effectiveness. Furthermore, self-hypnosis provides individuals with the means to regain control over their relationship with food.

TECHNIQUES FOR REDUCING CRAVINGS THROUGH SELF-HYPNOSIS

Self-hypnosis can be a good way of controlling cravings. Through visual imagery and self-hypnosis scripts designed to target specific triggers, self-hypnosis is an extremely effective method for curbing food desires and cravings. Visualize mindful eating—enjoying every bite slowly before moving on to smaller portions if necessary. Self-hypnosis can provide an anchor like thumb and finger pressure that will allow you to regain control if cravings arise. Develop a practice routine of self-hypnosis to optimize its effectiveness. Self-hypnosis can help satisfy cravings by using relaxation techniques and personalized suggestions, including progressive muscle relaxation with deep breathing to reduce stress-induced cravings. Recorded sessions for on-the-spot assistance complete your arsenal for successfully controlling cravings.

CHAPTER 7: TRANSFORMING BODY IMAGE THROUGH SELF-HYPNOSIS

Challenging Negative Body Image Beliefs

Negative body image beliefs, often stemming from social pressures, can significantly erode self-esteem and confidence levels. Self-hypnosis offers an effective method for challenging these misconceptions and shifting them. It provides individuals with an effective tool for uncovering negative beliefs and challenging irrational thoughts; visually enhancing self-image while relieving anxiety related to self-criticism are among the many goals achieved through its practice. Consistent practice reinforces new, positive beliefs for those struggling with entrenched issues. Self-hypnosis provides an avenue for building healthier self-esteem and body confidence, thus contributing to both overall well-being and personal growth.

CREATING POSITIVE AFFIRMATIONS FOR BODY ACCEPTANCE

Effective affirmation techniques combined with regular self-hypnosis can transform body perception. Craft affirmation statements that are specific, positive, and present-focused, ensuring they feel believable and crafted specifically for you. Speaking in first person may increase emotional resonance while keeping statements concise can make recalling them easier during self-hypnosis sessions. Recording and playing back your voice or placing affirmation cards around reinforces their message throughout your day and helps promote an accepting and loving attitude toward body image that ultimately fosters increased self-esteem and confidence.

PRACTICING SELF-HYPNOSIS FOR BODY CONFIDENCE AND SELF-ESTEEM

Self-hypnosis techniques are a powerful tool for enhancing your body's confidence and self-esteem by rewiring your subconscious mind. Through visualization exercises and guided imagery, you can construct a mental portrait of yourself brimming with confidence and high self-esteem. Regular self-hypnosis practice serves as the nurturing ground for a more constructive mindset, fostering a robust basis of self-belief and self-acceptance. This practice empowers you to shatter self-doubt, replace it with self-assurance, and manifest the positive self-image you desire. With dedication, self-hypnosis can transform your perception of yourself, bolstering your confidence and self-esteem for lasting change.

CHAPTER 8: ESTABLISHING HEALTHY HABITS AND MINDSET

Creating New Positive Habits Through Self-Hypnosis

Creating new positive habits through self-hypnosis is a transformative journey. To embark on this path, begin by setting clear, present-tense goals for the habits you wish to cultivate, such as "I am a healthier eater" or "I consistently exercise."

In a quiet, distraction-free space, relax your body and mind with deep breaths and close your eyes. Construct a series of succinct, powerful affirmations that align with your goals. Visualization is key; vividly imagine yourself successfully practicing these habits and savoring their benefits.

Induce a hypnotic state through techniques like progressive muscle relaxation or counting backward.

While in this relaxed state, repeat your affirmations, letting them penetrate your subconscious. Create a trigger word or action that you can use in your daily life to reinforce your self-hypnosis.

Consistency is crucial. Dedicate a few minutes daily to self-hypnosis and maintain unwavering self-belief. Record your progress in a journal, embracing setbacks as part of the process. Patience is your ally; trust the process and watch your positive habits become an integral part of your life.

REPROGRAMMING THE SUBCONSCIOUS MIND FOR LONG-TERM SUCCESS

The subconscious mind wields immense power, containing approximately 95% of our thoughts, feelings, and memories. Dr. Bruce Lipton notes its staggering influence, being a million times more potent than our conscious mind, capable of processing 11 million bits of information per second. Reprogramming the subconscious for lasting success requires distinguishing it from the conscious mind. The conscious mind handles awareness, emotions, thoughts, and physical sensations, while the subconscious shapes our behaviors (Pierson, 2022). To harness this power, visualization paints a clear path to goals alongside affirming mantras that conquer fears. Regularly vocalizing goals reinforces commitment. By filtering thoughts and dispelling fear and doubt, the subconscious can be cultivated for positive habits, aligning with Carl Gustav Jung's insight: "Until you make the unconscious conscious, it will direct your life."

USING SELF-HYPNOSIS FOR MOTIVATION AND CONSISTENCY

Self-hypnosis offers a potent avenue for bolstering your motivation and ensuring consistency in pursuing your goals. Through this powerful technique, you can effectively substitute unproductive subconscious thought patterns with more constructive ones. By inducing a tranquil yet focused mental state, you pave the way for a profound transformation in your mindset. In terms of motivation, self-hypnosis helps you reprogram your inner dialogue, instilling a resolute sense of purpose and enthusiasm for your objectives. It empowers you to tap into your deepest desires and channel them toward productive actions. On the consistency front, self-hypnosis assists in establishing a routine by enhancing your self-discipline and diminishing distractions. This practice not only sharpens your concentration but also reinforces your commitment to daily tasks. In essence, self-hypnosis is a dynamic tool that can empower you to access your inner drive, bolstering both motivation and consistency on your path to success.

CHAPTER 9: SELF-HYPNOSIS FOR STRESS AND EMOTIONAL WELL-BEING

Understanding the Connection Between Stress and Weight

Stress and weight gain are inextricably interlinked due to their complex hormonal impact on our bodies. Cortisol, released as a reactionary response from stress hormones, may increase appetite, particularly for high-caloric foods, while encouraging fat storage around abdominal regions. Stressful events may also disrupt sleep patterns and contribute to insomnia, something linked with weight gain. It's not uncommon for stress to trigger emotional eating, as people use food as an emotional release valve when experiencing difficulties or negative feelings; physical activity decreases, and unhealthy coping methods like smoking, drinking alcohol, or using drugs may worsen weight issues further, so managing stress levels effectively is crucial to keeping our weight under control and our overall well-being intact.

USING SELF-HYPNOSIS FOR RELAXATION AND STRESS REDUCTION

Self-hypnosis can be learned and practiced independently with only minimal guidance required, making it a practical and cost-effective solution to effective stress relief strategies.

Before beginning self-hypnosis, find a relaxing environment—whether sitting or lying down—in which to begin your practice. After setting an intention—whether reducing stress, building confidence, or facing fears—begin taking deep, slow breaths through both nostrils before exhaling through the mouth for best results. This should calm both mind and body before moving on to other steps of the hypnosis journey.

Progressive muscle relaxation begins by stretching each muscle group briefly before relaxing it—from your toes up. Try closing your eyes and visualizing an inviting scene involving all senses; create positive affirmations related to your goal slowly but confidently; or simply say slow and meaningful affirmations related to them out loud.

Hypnotic induction helps create a deep state of relaxation through counting or relaxing phrases; deepening techniques may include visualizing stairs descending or an elevator going downwards.

Within this elevated state, use vivid imagery to visualize success. Reiterate positive suggestions before awakening by counting up from 1-5 or using awakening phrases. Reflect upon the experience and practice regularly to strengthen positive suggestions while deepening relaxation.

TECHNIQUES FOR ENHANCING EMOTIONAL WELL-BEING THROUGH SELF-HYPNOSIS

Self-hypnosis is a holistic technique to enhance mental well-being by nurturing mindfulness, relaxation, and psychological fortitude. Self-hypnosis is putting yourself in a highly focused and suggestible state. By embracing this method and integrating it into our daily routines, we can better control our reactions to food, foster optimism, and lead a sustainable, mentally sound lifestyle. Mental health significantly impacts weight management, as unfavorable feelings often trigger unhealthy eating habits that affect one's weight. Through practices like visualization, positive confirmations, and behavior reprogramming, we can reshape our connection with food and become more aware of our emotions and factors that can influence eating habits.

Accessing our subconscious allows us to initiate positive transformations while reframing pessimistic thought patterns. Self-hypnosis may even boost self-esteem by substituting negative self-talk with constructive convictions that amplify one's self-worth. Effective management of anger and irritability involves training our minds to respond calmly to triggers, and desensitizing emotional reactions is vital for overcoming fears or phobias. Self-hypnosis offers numerous therapeutic benefits, aiding in coping with grief and loss, enhancing relaxation and sleep patterns, pain control, breaking undesirable habits, building self-assurance, and strengthening mental resilience.

CHAPTER 10: OPTIMIZING SLEEP WITH SELF-HYPNOSIS

The Impact of Sleep on Weight Management

Sleep is vital to weight management. A lack of quality rest disrupts hormone balance in your body, altering appetite and metabolism—as evidenced by increased hunger hormone ghrelin and decreased leptin (which signals fullness). When this occurs, we often tend to overeat high-calorie and sugary foods more readily due to reduced leptin signaling fullness, leading to overeating as a result. Furthermore, quality rest is crucial in controlling blood sugar levels and insulin sensitivity—when this process becomes impaired it leads to weight gain as well as risk for type 2 diabetes—making prioritizing quality sleep just as crucial in maintaining a healthy body. Maintaining a healthy weight requires prioritizing quality rest as much as maintaining regular nutrition and physical exercise regimens.

USING SELF-HYPNOSIS FOR BETTER SLEEP AND INSOMNIA

Self-hypnosis provides various techniques to enhance sleep quality and address insomnia by leveraging the power of your mind. By following these steps, you can induce relaxation through self-hypnosis for a peaceful mindset and better sleep.

- Find a quiet, comfortable space.

- Choose a comfy position.

- Practice controlled breathing.

- Select a self-hypnosis method.

- Use guided imagery or muscle relaxation.

- Use positive affirmations.

- Allocate 15-20 minutes for practice.

Self-hypnosis can aid sleep disorders like sleep apnea and restless leg syndrome, offering a noninvasive alternative to traditional treatments.

PRACTICES FOR ENHANCING SLEEP HYGIENE THROUGH SELF-HYPNOSIS

Enhancing the quality of your sleep involves mixing several essential sleep hygiene practices with the application of self-hypnosis. To begin, adhering to a consistent sleep schedule—where you retire to bed and rise at the same times each day—provides stability to your body's internal clock, which complements the relaxation achieved through self-hypnosis. Creating a sleep-conducive environment is equally vital, as a cool, dark, and quiet room encourages undisturbed rest. Minimizing exposure to screens and stimulating activities before bedtime is crucial since the blue light emitted by electronic devices can disrupt your circadian rhythms. Moreover, abstaining from caffeine, heavy meals, alcohol, and nicotine in the evening can further minimize sleep disturbances, making self-hypnosis more effective. To build on this foundation, consider reducing noise and light disturbances, which can be achieved through earplugs, blackout curtains, or white noise machines. Additionally, ensure a comfortable sleep environment with a supportive mattress and cozy bedding. Developing bedtime routines that incorporate self-hypnosis, such as relaxation exercises and guided imagery, can be highly beneficial. For example, you might engage in deep breathing exercises and visualize a peaceful, serene place as part of your pre-sleep ritual, gradually incorporating self-hypnosis techniques. By amalgamating these sleep hygiene practices with self-hypnosis and personalized bedtime routines, we can craft a comprehensive strategy to optimize sleep quality.

CHAPTER 11: MAINTAINING WEIGHT LOSS WITH SELF-HYPNOSIS

Preventing Weight Regain Through Self-Hypnosis

Combining self-hypnosis techniques with effective weight maintenance strategies can offer a comprehensive approach to sustaining a healthy weight. Set realistic goals and instill a sense of belief in your capacity to achieve and preserve your ideal weight.

Self-hypnosis helps incorporate lifestyle changes by reducing stress and enhancing receptivity to positive suggestions about healthier eating and regular exercise. It reinforces the habit of controlling unhealthy food cravings and visualizing satisfaction with smaller portions.

Use self-hypnosis to boost motivation for consistent physical activity. Visualize enjoying exercise, reaching fitness goals with ease, and staying committed. Self-hypnosis promotes self-awareness, reinforces tracking food and exercise, and reminds you to stay adequately hydrated.

Cultivate mindfulness during meals through self-hypnosis, savoring each bite, and recognizing fullness cues. Manage emotional triggers for overeating via self-hypnosis, finding healthier coping strategies for stress and emotions.

Enhance your support system with self-hypnosis, visualizing the encouragement and sharing of goals and challenges with friends and family. Maintain regular self-hypnosis check-ins and treat setbacks as learning opportunities, using visualization to stay positive.

Self-hypnosis can complement professional guidance, reinforcing motivation and receptivity. By combining self-hypnosis with these strategies, you can strengthen your commitment to a lasting, healthy lifestyle. This synergy can significantly boost your ability to prevent regaining weight.

DEVELOPING MINDSET AND HABITS FOR WEIGHT MAINTENANCE

Losing weight is a significant achievement yet maintaining it can be a formidable challenge. It requires more than sheer willpower and occasional dieting; it necessitates a profound transformation of your mindset and the development of lasting habits. Fostering a positive, enduring mindset, cultivating self-discipline, and embracing health-conscious lifestyle practices all play vital roles in the sustained success of weight management.

THE SIGNIFICANCE OF MINDSET

- Begin your journey with a constructive outlook. View setbacks as opportunities for growth, not failures.

- A resilient mindset enables recovery from setbacks and prevents an all-or-nothing mentality.

BUILDING SELF-DISCIPLINE

- Establish specific, attainable short-term and long-term objectives for weight maintenance.

- Consistency is key. Create a structured routine that includes regular exercise and a balanced diet.

- Keep records of your food intake and physical activity to maintain accountability and gain insights into your habits.

- Rely on friends, family, or a weight-loss group for motivation and accountability.

ADOPTING HEALTHY LIFESTYLE PRACTICES

- Maintain a diverse, portion-controlled diet, avoiding extreme restrictions.

- Include enjoyable physical activities as part of your daily life for both cardiovascular and strength training.

- Prioritize 7-9 hours of quality sleep, which is crucial for managing hunger hormones and making wise food choices.

- Practice stress-reduction techniques, such as mindfulness or yoga, to prevent emotional eating.

- Acknowledge non-scale achievements, like enhanced energy levels and better-fitting clothes, in addition to scale progress.

It's not a linear path, but your dedication will bring lasting success to your quest for a healthier, happier you.

CONTINUOUS SELF-HYPNOSIS PRACTICE FOR LONG-TERM SUCCESS

Consistency in self-hypnosis is pivotal for effective weight control. Rooted in the power of the mind, this practice thrives on regular and systematic engagement. It reinforces positive behaviors and beliefs concerning body and mind states. Engaging in self-hypnosis for weight management establishes a structured routine that counters the temptations and fluctuations that often lead to weight gain. It ensures the subconscious mind continually receives positive reinforcement, fortifying the determination to make healthier choices and maintain an ideal weight.

By infusing self-hypnosis techniques into everyday activities, we unlock our full subconscious potential, fostering enduring change. When self-hypnosis becomes as ingrained as daily hygiene or the morning coffee ritual, it embeds positive suggestions and intentions into daily life. This integration promotes the ability to overcome challenges, reduce stress, and achieve personal objectives. Over time, self-hypnosis shapes thought processes and behaviors, making it an invaluable tool for personal growth.

To maintain motivation, it's vital to set clear, achievable goals and revisit them regularly to maintain focus. Building a supportive network can provide valuable encouragement. When facing hurdles, viewing setbacks as opportunities to learn and adjust our approach is essential. Flexibility is key, as weight management is a dynamic process. Different phases may require customized techniques, such as modifying self-hypnosis scripts to address evolving objectives or integrating new strategies to overcome plateaus. Adaptation, motivation, and perseverance are the keys to a healthier, happier lifestyle.

CHAPTER 12: CASE STUDIES: REAL-LIFE SUCCESS STORIES

Interviews With Individuals Who Used Self-Hypnosis for Weight Loss

Within our exploration of self-hypnosis for weight loss, we've encountered remarkable individuals who harnessed this transformative technique to reshape their lives. Julie Evans, Sarah, Lisa, and a courageous 35-year-old woman generously shared their motivational journeys.

Julie Evans, burdened by the weight of past diet attempts, found herself intrigued by hypnosis. Skepticism didn't deter her from trying a hypnosis gastric bypass, which revolutionized her approach to food. Portion control and a newfound craving for healthy choices became her allies (Schmidt, 2014).

Sarah's path was paved with self-doubt and food addiction. With self-hypnosis, she reprogrammed her mental landscape, dismantling the walls of self-sabotage. Her 144-

pound weight loss stands as a testament to her dedication and the power of mind over matter (*My Weight-Loss Success with Hypnotherapy*, n.d.).

Lisa confronted emotional eating and skepticism head-on. She immersed herself in self-hypnosis, peeling back layers to reveal the roots of her emotional eating. The result? Remarkable weight loss and a healthier relationship with nourishment.

Our 35-year-old heroine embarked on a dual quest: shedding weight and conquering a fear of motorways. Self-hypnosis became her guiding star, illuminating a path to transformation. In 11 months, her goal weight of 9 stone 10 pounds became a reality, while her fear of motorways faded into insignificance (Glover, 2015).

HIGHLIGHTING THEIR JOURNEY, CHALLENGES, AND OUTCOMES

Their stories are threads woven into the tapestry of challenges, obstacles, and achievements. Julie conquered skepticism, Sarah grappled with self-doubt, Lisa faced emotional eating, and the 35-year-old woman tackled fear. Through self-hypnosis, they found the tools to rewrite their narratives.

LESSONS AND INSPIRATION FROM THEIR EXPERIENCES

These stories convey profound lessons. First, self-hypnosis is a versatile tool that adapts to diverse needs. Second, it requires confronting skepticism and self-doubt. Lisa's journey illuminates the importance of addressing the root causes of emotional eating. Lastly, embracing self-hypnosis can lead to remarkable outcomes.

These individuals' journeys exemplify the extraordinary possibilities of self-hypnosis in weight loss and personal transformation. As you embark on your own path, remember that self-hypnosis can be your steadfast companion, offering the tools to reshape your relationship with food and fears. Their triumphs are living proof that change is within reach for those who dare to dream and take the first step.

CHAPTER 13: ADDRESSING COMMON CONCERNS AND MISCONCEPTIONS

Safety and Ethical Considerations

While generally considered safe, self-hypnosis for weight loss demands a responsible approach to safety. Key considerations include:

- Seeking counsel from a certified hypnotherapist or health care expert is advisable. They can customize the self-hypnosis process and offer ongoing support.

- Steer clear of self-hypnosis practices promising extreme or unattainable results. Techniques that advocate self-deprivation or negative self-suggestions should be eschewed, as they may harm your mental and physical well-being.

- Always engage in self-hypnosis with full awareness of the process, potential outcomes, and associated risks. This preserves your autonomy and ensures a controlled experience.

Ethical considerations are equally critical. The practice of self-hypnosis for weight loss should align with ethical standards:

- Self-hypnosis should empower individuals to make their own choices and decisions without coercion or manipulation.

- Confidentiality: When seeking guidance from a hypnotherapist or counselor, they must uphold confidentiality and safeguard your privacy.

- Employ self-hypnosis techniques that promote well-being and avert harm. Steer clear of practices that could induce psychological distress or unhealthy behaviors.

MYTHS AND MISCONCEPTIONS SURROUNDING SELF-HYPNOSIS

Debunking common myths and misconceptions is pivotal for a clear understanding of self-hypnosis for weight loss:

- Self-hypnosis is not about controlling minds. It's a collaborative process where you retain control and can terminate it at your discretion.

- Special abilities are unnecessary for self-hypnosis. It's a skill acquired through practice and guidance.

- Self-hypnosis serves self-improvement, not entertainment like stage hypnosis. Goals differ, with self-hypnosis focused on personal objectives, such as weight loss.

EXPLAINING THE LIMITATIONS OF SELF-HYPNOSIS

Recognizing the limitations of self-hypnosis is vital:

- Self-hypnosis is not a magical, instant solution for weight loss. It necessitates dedication, consistency, and time, with results varying from person to person.

- Self-hypnosis may not be universally effective. Individual responses to hypnosis differ, with some being more receptive than others.

- Self-hypnosis thrives as part of a broader weight-loss approach. It's most effective when combined with healthy lifestyle changes like balanced nutrition and regular exercise.

Responsible self-hypnosis mandates a commitment to safety, ethical conduct, and understanding its limitations. By dispelling misconceptions and practicing self-hypnosis judiciously, we can employ this tool to realize weight-loss goals while safeguarding our well-being and autonomy.

CONCLUSION

EMPOWERING YOURSELF FOR LASTING WEIGHT LOSS

As we reach the end of this incredible adventure, let's come together once more for an introspection session. You have learned much about self-hypnosis as an effective weight-loss strategy; now let's assess all that we've accomplished so far and discuss where our journey leads next.

RECAP OF SELF-HYPNOSIS PRINCIPLES AND TECHNIQUES

Think back to the potent self-hypnosis techniques you've assimilated: the ability to vividly visualize, the art of effective suggestion, and the transformative impact of affirmations. These aren't just concepts anymore; they're your secret weapons in crafting the body and life you desire.

ENCOURAGEMENT AND MOTIVATION FOR ONGOING PRACTICE

Along this journey, you've faced challenges and moments when your willpower wavered. It's crucial to acknowledge that these hurdles are part of the path and each time you've persevered, you've grown stronger. With consistent self-hypnosis practice, you'll turn those challenges into stepping stones. Keep your motivation burning bright, and don't let any obstacle dim your determination.

FINAL THOUGHTS AND CALL TO ACTION FOR READERS

Your mind is the most incredible tool at your disposal, and it's capable of astonishing things. So, we implore you to keep harnessing self-hypnosis to fuel your weight-loss dreams. This journey is an ongoing adventure, and the path ahead is rich with promise.

You've learned the importance of setting attainable goals and nurturing them with patience, much like a gardener cultivating a thriving garden. Mindful eating, listening to your body's cues, and choosing nourishing whole foods are your keys to success. Habits form over time, and your consistency is the cornerstone of lasting change.

Reprogramming your subconscious mind for enduring success is no small feat, but you've got it down. You know how to seamlessly integrate self-hypnosis into your daily life, and you've witnessed real-life stories of individuals who've experienced incredible transformations through these practices.

"Losing Weight Through Self-Hypnosis" has been your

guide, but you have been the hero of this journey. These principles and techniques aren't just tools; they're the very essence of your transformation. Keep moving forward with unshakable determination, and you will realize the enduring weight loss success you've always envisioned. Your journey is a continuous adventure, teeming with boundless possibilities. Maintain faith in yourself, and let your journey continue to astound you.

REFERENCES

Glover, S. (2015, May 5). *A real weight-loss success story.* Hypnotherapy Directory. https://www.hypnotherapy-directory.org.uk/memberarticles/a-real-weight-loss-success-story

Lehrer, P. (2022). My Life in HRV Biofeedback Research. *Applied Psychophysiology and Biofeedback.* https://doi.org/10.1007/s10484-022-09535-5

Litwic-Kaminska, K., Kotyśko, M., Pracki, T., Wiłkość-Dębczyńska, M., & Stankiewicz, B. (2022). The Effect of Autogenic Training in a Form of Audio Recording on Sleep Quality and Physiological Stress Reactions of University Athletes—Pilot Study. *International Journal of Environmental Research and Public Health, 19*(23), 16043. https://doi.org/10.3390/ijerph192316043

My Weight-Loss Success With Hypnotherapy. (n.d.). My Weigh Less. https://myweighless.com/weight-loss-success-stories/sarahs-weight-loss-success-story/

Oliveira, J. (n.d.). *The Psychology of Successful Habits: Harnessing Routines for Positive Change.* Balance & Bliss. https://bblissmagazine.blogspot.com/2023/09/the-psychology-of-successful-habits.html

Palsson, O. S., Kekecs, Z., De Benedittis, G., Moss, D., Elkins,

G. R., Terhune, D. B., Varga, K., Shenefelt, P. D., & Whorwell, P. J. (2023). Current Practices, Experiences, and Views in Clinical Hypnosis: Findings of an International Survey. *International Journal of Clinical and Experimental Hypnosis*, 1–23. https://doi.org/10.1080/00207144.2023.2183862

Parvez, H. (2014, August 12). *Belief systems as subconscious programs* . PsychMechanics. https://www.psychmechanics.com/belief-systems-programs-of-subconscious/

Pellegrini, M., Carletto, S., Scumaci, E., Ponzo, V., Ostacoli, L., & Bo, S. (2021). The Use of Self-Help Strategies in Obesity Treatment. A Narrative Review Focused on Hypnosis and Mindfulness. *Current Obesity Reports*. https://doi.org/10.1007/s13679-021-00443-z

Pierson, J. (2022, November). *The Power of the Subconscious Mind*. RearchGate. https://www.researchgate.net/publication/365211107_The_Power_of_the_Subconscious_Mind

Randall, C. (2022, January 2). *Hypnosis for motivation.* Hypnotherapy Directory. https://www.hypnotherapy-directory.org.uk/blog/2022/01/02/hypnosis-for-motivation

Russell, K. L., Rodman, H. R., & Pak, V. M. (2023). Sleep insufficiency, circadian rhythms, and metabolomics: the connection between metabolic and sleep disorders. *Sleep and Breathing*. https://doi.org/10.1007/s11325-023-02828-x

Sarrafi-Zadeh, S. (2012). Nutritional Modulators of Sleep Disorders. *The Open Nutraceuticals Journal*, 5(1), 1–14.

https://doi.org/10.2174/1876396001205010001

Schmidt, C. (2014, August 18). *Hypnosis helped her lose 140 pounds*. CNN. https://edition.cnn.com/2014/08/18/health/weight-loss-julie-evans/index.html

Weight Loss Success Stories - Weight Loss Hypnosis. (n.d.). The Weightloss Coach. https://www.saweightlosshypnosis.com.au/SuccessStories?r_done=1

Williamson, A. (2019). What is hypnosis and how might it work? *Palliative Care: Research and Treatment, 12*(1), 117822421982658. https://doi.org/10.1177/1178224219826581

Young, A. (2021, February 1). *Reprogramming Your Subconscious Mind: A Step-By-Step Guide*. Rainmakers. https://gorainmakers.com/2021/02/01/reprogramming-your-subconscious-mind-a-step-by-step-guide/